DIABETES HANDBOOK

Diabetes is a long-term metabolic disease in which the body is unable to control blood-sugar levels. The food we eat turns into glucose (sugar) during the metabolic process and the normal body's pancreas produces insulin that allows the body to use the glucose for energy and muscle by activating the cells to accept the glucose. The diabetic's pancreas does not produce enough insulin, or produces no insulin at all.

Diabetes can be managed and controlled with insulin, exercise, weight control, and frequent blood tests. If managed properly the diabetic can live a long life with few complications. Some diabetics have a fatalistic view of the disease because most diabetes publications only discuss the negative effects. This booklet shows how to control diabetes and maintain a positive attitude and a positive outlook on life.

Management of diabetes is up to the individual – there are no magic formulas. The tools are available for diabetes management. Insulin injections solve the pancreas problem, and blood-test devices are available for frequent blood testing. All the diabetic has to do is use these tools to manage the disease.

Diabetes has been around forever. The disease was described as "too great emptying of the urine" in a 1500 BC Egyptian manuscript. In 250 BC, the Greeks discovered two types of diabetes, and even though today's classification as Type 1 and Type 2 was not identified as such, the difference between people who died of the disease and those who suffered with the disease, but did not die was obvious.

Even though diabetes does not receive as much publicity as AIDs and breast cancer, the disease kills more people than these two illnesses combined. Diabetes kills over 1.5 million people in America every year, and the cost of diabetes treatment is greater than $250 billion annually. This figure does not include approximately $175 billion in hospital costs, and $75 billion in indirect medical costs such as absenteeism from work.

There are a number of diabetes publications, but it is difficult to find a small handbook that describes the disease in an easy-to-read format, and includes specific data on sugar levels, daily problems, and solutions. The need for frequent blood tests is discussed along with the need for insulin corrections. Only diabetics know of the daily problems, and these issues are covered. One problem not covered in existing publications is the diabetic's refusal to accept a sugar supplement for hypoglycemia because the individual does not recognize or accept the symptoms.

WHAT IS DIABETES

Diabetes is an incurable metabolic disease resulting from the body's inability to process blood sugar. Surprisingly, the exact cause of diabetes is unknown. The accepted causes are genetics and lifestyle such as excess weight, and in some cases, a virus causes the immune system to attack the pancreas and kill its insulin making capability.

When the body digests food, carbohydrates are reduced to glucose (sugar), and the liver processes fats and protein into glucose. The normal body's pancreas reacts by producing a chemical called insulin, which allows the body to use the sugar for energy and muscle by triggering the cells to accept sugar. The diabetic's pancreas produces either no insulin, or an insufficient amount of insulin to process the sugar. In some cases, the body cells reject the sugar.

There are over 30 million diabetics in America, which is approximately 10% of the population, and more than 380 million worldwide. The number of diabetics is increasing dramatically – in the last decade the number of people living with diabetes increased over 50%.

It wasn't until the nineteenth century that scientists discovered that patients who died of diabetes had a damaged pancreas. In 1869, a German student, Paul Langerhaus, discovered that the beta cells in the pancreas produced insulin. However, another 50 years went by before insulin became available for diabetes treatment.

TYPES OF DIABETES

· Type 1: The diabetic's pancreas produces no insulin, and daily injections of insulin are required to keep the person alive. Type 1 diabetes is sometimes caused by certain viral infections that mistakenly cause the body's immune system to attack the pancreas and kill the insulin making capability of the beta cells.

· Type 2: The diabetic's pancreas does not produce enough insulin to handle blood sugar. The exact cause of Type 2 is also unknown, but again genetics is thought to be a causal factor along with excess weight.

· Type 3: Gestational diabetes occurs during pregnancy and is sometimes called Type 3 diabetes. Most gestational diabetes goes away after birth, but it does put the individual at higher risk of becoming diabetic.

· Type 4: Prediabetes is when the blood sugar is higher than normal, but not high enough to be classified as a Type 2 .

If food is not processed with insulin, the sugar does not go into the cells and just passes through the body. The sugar is eventually excreted in the urine. As a result, the body cells do not receive the energy and muscle to function properly. If the body produces no insulin the individual is a Type 1 diabetic, the body loses weight, wastes away, and the diabetic usually dies in a few years (or less) without insulin.

The second type of diabetes (Type 2) is less severe. The Type 2 diabetic's pancreas produces insulin, but the amount is insufficient to process all the blood sugar. Some diabetics also have the problem of cells rejecting insulin. The treatment for Type 2 diabetics includes a strict diet, exercise, and medication (not normally insulin) that squeezes more insulin from the pancreas. Few Type 2 diabetics adhere to a strict diet and fail to exercise properly. This results in high blood-sugar levels and often leads to hyperglycemia.

For centuries, there was no medication (insulin) for Type 1 diabetics, and people with the disease continuously lost weight since the blood sugar passed through the body and they simply died. In most cases, the Type 1 diabetic was unaware of the cause of the disease since there was little medical research and information. Type 1 diabetes was formerly known as the "wasting disease."

WHAT IS INSULIN

Although diabetes has been recognized for over 3500 years, successful treatment of the disease was not developed until 1921 when Dr. Frederick Banting developed insulin. Before the discovery of insulin, the treatment for diabetes involved a strict diet. The diet treatment only added a few years to the diabetic's life, and in some cases, people died of starvation because of the rigorous diet – a terrible way to die. Diabetes was known as the "wasting disease" since diabetics simply wasted away and died. Few present-day Type 1 diabetics, who are fortunate to have insulin for treatment, appreciate that if they had been born a hundred years ago they would be dead. The development of insulin finally allowed people with diabetes to live an almost normal life.

Insulin is a protein hormone produced by the beta cells in the human pancreas that regulates the blood sugar. The chemical allows the body to use glucose from food by triggering the body's cells to accept sugar. When food is digested the blood sugar rises, and the body signals the pancreas to release insulin into the blood stream. The insulin then triggers the cells in the body to absorb sugar for energy. Insulin is the key that unlocks the cells permitting the sugar to enter the cells and provide energy and muscle. Insulin also helps store sugar in the liver for emergencies such as exercise.

The body is an amazing machine but sometimes malfunctions occur. Several viruses are suspected to be associated with diabetes including mumps and German Measles. When the viruses cause the immune system to kill the beta cells of the pancreas the person becomes an insulin-dependent diabetic (Type 1), normally within a few months. In other cases, the pancreas does not produce enough insulin, or the cells do not accept the insulin, and the individual becomes a non-insulin-dependent diabetic, which is classified as Type 2.

Dr. Frederick Banting was an orthopedic surgeon and worked in Toronto's Hospital for Sick Children. The sight of children dying of diabetes at an early age prompted him to pursue a cure for diabetes. Research had shown that the body's pancreas produced a chemical called insulin, and it was believed that insulin controlled the metabolism of sugar. Dr. Banting started working with animal pancreas in an attempt to develop insulin. After successfully developing insulin, Banting and his associate Professor Macleod were awarded the Nobel Prize in 1923.

Without insulin, glucose is not transferred into the cells, and passes through the body in the blood stream. The glucose is then excreted in the urine. The thirst symptom causes the diabetic to drink an excessive amount of fluids. Hence, the Egyptian description of "too great emptying of the urine."

The development of insulin by Dr. Banting was a historic event. Before the insulin treatment diabetics just died of the disease since the body did not receive the necessary energy to survive. Banting and his assistant Charles Best began experimenting with dog pancreas, and were able to extract insulin. After experimenting with animals, Banting found that insulin corrected the blood sugar problem, and began injecting patients with insulin. The diabetes symptoms of high blood sugar, extreme thirst, and weight loss disappeared, and Frederick Banting had discovered a treatment for diabetes.

Eli Lilly and Company started producing insulin in 1923 for human use. The first insulin came from animal pancreas, but most of today's insulin is produced in laboratories by introducing a synthetic human gene into bacteria or yeast. Laboratory insulin has nearly the same effect on blood sugar as human insulin, but does have a faster onset and a shorter duration.

Companies have developed many (20) types of insulin since the 1920s and the insulins are suspended in fluids to permit taking insulin as a shot. A syringe, insulin pen, or insulin pump is required for insulin intake because the body's digestive system breaks down a pill before it can be absorbed into the blood stream. The strength of the many insulins is most commonly U-100, which has 100 units of insulin per millimeter of fluid.

The various types of insulin are classified by the time – element. There are rapid-term, short-term, intermediate-term, and long-term insulins, and the following are the specifics.

- Rapid-term insulin begins working in 15 minutes, peaks in 1 - 2 hours, and continues to work for four hours. Trade names are Humalog and Novolog.

- Short-term insulin begins working in 30 minutes, peaks in 2 - 3 hours, and continues to work for six hours. Trade names are Humulin R and Novilin R.

- Intermediate-term insulin begins in 1 – 2 hours, peaks in 4 – 8 hours, and continues to work for 12 – 18 hours. Trade names are Humulin N and Novilin N

- Long-term insulin begins working in 1 – 2 hours, peaks in 4 hours, and is constant for 24 hours. Trade names are Lantus Glargine and Levemir.

Type 1 diabetics normally take a rapid-term (4-hour) insulin to handle food at each meal, and a long-term (24-hour) insulin at night. The long-term insulin is required because the Type 1 diabetic's pancreas produces no insulin and insulin is required during the night. The diabetic must be aware that the long-term insulin can often cause low-blood sugar during the night and result in hypoglycemia. The individual must make sure the blood sugar is high enough (120 mg/gl) at bedtime to avoid hypoglycemia.

The amount of insulin to take is determined by testing blood sugar levels. Several test devices have been developed, and the test process requires the diabetic to prick his/her finger, place the blood on a test strip, and insert the strip into the test device. The first job for a Type 1 diabetic is to determine the amount of sugar handled by one unit of insulin.

The metabolism of each individual is unique; therefore, the effect of insulin is also unique. In my case, one unit of rapid-acting insulin handles 25 mg/dl of sugar. The diabetic must determine the exact amount of sugar handled by one unit of insulin in his/her body by testing several times and recording the data like a scientific experiment. This is a key statistic since it determines the amount of rapid-term insulin to be taken at meals. The sugar-level reading and the type and amount of food intake dictate the amount of insulin required.

Frequent blood testing two hours after meals will allow the diabetic to recognize the amount of insulin necessary to maintain blood sugar at the desired level of 100 mg/dl.

The amount of long-term insulin required is more difficult to determine, and the endocrinologist should be consulted. Again, the Type 1 diabetic should be aware of the danger of low-blood sugar (hypoglycemia), and make sure that the blood-sugar level is high enough at bedtime to avoid hypoglycemia. The amount of long-term insulin required is normally determined through trial-and-error testing.

CORRECTIONS

The Type 1 diabetic should make corrections during the day to assure that the blood sugar is under control. Frequent blood-sugar tests should be taken two hours after meals to check blood-sugar levels, and additional insulin should be taken if a correction is required. The blood-sugar level should be approximately 140 mg/dl two hours after a meal. If the reading is 200 mg/dl or higher, the diabetic must take more insulin. Since rapid-term insulin has a four-hour duration, there are two hours of insulin remaining from the prior shot. Overlap in insulin is a risk that must be avoided, so the diabetic should develop the correct amount of insulin required to meet the target blood sugar of 100 mg/dl. Trial-and-error testing is necessary to determine the insulin levels required for correction.

Diabetics are directed to measure food and calculate carbohydrate intake, but few do this with any degree of accuracy. Many diabetics eat their normal diet without regard to being diabetic. This is of course, wrong, but it occurs. This leads to poor control, and often results in hypoglycemia or hyperglycemia, which are the two major risks for diabetics.

Insulin-dependent diabetics' primary problem in controlling diabetes is to determine the amount of insulin required to meet the target level of 100mg/dl, and stay in the range between hypoglycemia (low blood sugar), and hyperglycemia (high blood sugar). Both low and high sugar levels are life-threatening.

The range between low and high sugar levels is small, with 65 mg/gl being the limit on the low side, and 240 mg/gl the limit on the high side. When 45 minutes of exercise on a treadmill burns 100 mg/gl of sugar, and a single candy bar can increase blood sugar by 100 mg/gl, the diabetic must recognize just how close sugar levels must be controlled. The 100 mg/dl is over 50% of the total range between the low and high blood sugar limits. The individual is faced with the task of attempting to duplicate the body's pancreas in the processing of food intake, and this is not an easy job.

HYPOGLYCEMIA

Hypoglycemia is a low blood sugar condition that can cause dangerous problems that are life threatening. The diabetic can become unconscious, or fall into a coma. The symptoms of hypoglycemia are listed on page 16, but the diabetic sometimes feels no symptom and is unable to recognize the problem. The onset of hypoglycemia is sudden, and if no symptoms occur, the diabetic is unable to react to the problem. If the blood sugar falls to 35 mg/dl or lower, and the diabetic does not feel a symptom, the individual becomes unconscious, and it is necessary for someone to call an emergency medical technician (EMT) to administer an IV with sugar to bring the person back to normal. If the diabetic feels no symptoms, the individual often refuses to accept sugar to correct the situation. This problem is not mentioned in diabetes publications because only diabetics who have experienced the refusal problem know about the condition. In extreme situations, the diabetic refuses to open his/her mouth to accept a sugar supplement.

It is important that the diabetic tell family, friends, and business associates about the hypoglycemic symptoms of profuse sweating, difficulty in walking, slurred speech, and confusion so they can help. Some of these symptoms are similar to drunkenness, so it is important to make friends aware of the hypoglycemia situation.

Hypoglycemia is extremely dangerous if the diabetic suffers the condition while driving a vehicle because the individual is unable to think clearly and certainly in no condition to drive. All diabetics should test their blood sugar level before driving a vehicle, and this test requirement is a cardinal rule. The blood test equipment (which is a small unit) should always be available. If any hypoglycemia symptoms such as profuse sweating occur while driving a vehicle, the diabetic must immediately pull the vehicle to the side of the road, and take a sugar supplement. A can or bottle of Coke is the easy solution for a sugar supplement because a few swallows of Coke raises the blood sugar immediately.

The difference between the low and high sugar level limits is less than 200 mg/dl. If the sugar level is 150 mg/dl, two hours of exercise can reduce the blood sugar level to the low sugar level limit, and two candy bars can raise blood sugar levels to the high sugar level limit. The diabetic has very little room between the low and high limits, and must be very careful. This close tolerance between hypoglycemia and hyperglycemia is not covered in diabetic publications, but it certainly is something to be aware of to manage diabetes properly. The diabetic should be aware of the dangers of hypoglycemia because the condition can be life threatening. Even if the diabetic catches the problem before becoming unconscious, the symptoms are embarrassing and dangerous.

For some unknown reason the body signals hypoglycemia more strongly than hyperglycemia. The symptoms of hypoglycemia occur suddenly (when they occur), and the diabetic is painfully aware that something is wrong. However, the symptoms of hyperglycemia occur some time after the sugar level is too high, and are not as dramatic as the hypoglycemia symptoms. Hyperglycemia is a hidden danger because the body does not signal any immediate symptoms.

Once the Type 1 individual recognizes the symptoms of hyperglycemia, he/she can immediately take insulin to bring the sugar level down. However, this is a problem for Type 2 diabetics if they are not on insulin, and hyperglycemia often continues for long periods.

The normal glucose level is approximately 100 mg/dl. If the blood-glucose level falls below 65 mg/dl brain efficiency declines, and if it falls below 50 mg/dl, hypoglycemia occurs with dangerous symptoms and side effects. The diabetic must not allow the sugar level fall much below 100 mg/d to assure that the hypoglycemic condition is avoided.

The body often reacts to hypoglycemia with intense symptoms and the individual is acutely aware that something is wrong. The onset of hypoglycemia is sudden and the individual has little time to correct the problem.

SYMPTOMS OF HYPOGLYCEMIA

· Decrease in brain function – unable to think clearly
· Profuse sweating
· Impaired judgement, confusion, abnormal thinking
· Slurred speech and difficulty speaking
· General motor problems – difficulty walking
· Impaired vision. When the blood sugar is below 60 the diabetic often sees rings similar to doughnuts which indicate hypoglycemia. This is often the first indication of low-blood sugar. Diabetes publications have not reported this symptom, but Type 1 diabetics recognize the doughnuts as the first sign of hypoglycemia.
· Personality change – often aggressive traits occur
· Unconsciousness and sometimes a coma
· Extreme hunger
    · The body reads the low sugar problem and demands sugar. This demand for food is unbelievably high and difficult to control. The body system does a great job telling the individual that blood sugar is low and that it is imperative that food is taken to solve the problem. The diabetic responds but normally eats too much because the drive to eat is so great. This solves the hypoglycemia problem but often creates a high blood sugar problem. The excess food intake also causes weight gain, which all diabetics must avoid.

Hypoglycemia often occurs when the diabetic attempts to control blood glucose too closely and takes too much insulin. It is ideal to control blood sugar closely but since there are so many variables in the equation, it is a difficult task. The result is often low blood sugar that requires additional food intake, which in most cases creates a high blood-sugar condition. The admirable attempt to control blood sugar actually results in just the opposite effect when low blood sugar occurs, and the diabetic is driven to eat too much food to correct the hypoglycemic condition and the result is hyperglycemia.

HYPERGLYCEMIA

Hyperglycemia is a condition caused by high blood sugar levels. While hypoglycemia sometimes gives an immediate reaction with profuse sweating and confusion, hyperglycemia is not readily noticeable. The symptoms of hyperglycemia are thirst, a dry mouth, and frequent urination because the body is telling the individual that the sugar level is too high, and gives the signal to drink liquids to rid the body of sugar. However, these symptoms occur some time after the high blood sugar reaches a dangerous level. Continuous hyperglycemia causes serious complications that cause painful, and sometimes fatal, consequences. The diabetic should test his/her blood sugar level whenever hyperglycemic symptoms occur. If the test shows a level of 240 mg/gl or higher, the individual is suffering from hyperglycemia, and the Type 1 diabetic must take insulin immediately. The condition is normally caused by insufficient insulin, although a cold or flu may have caused stress in the body and contributed to the high blood glucose level. Of course, excessive food intake or the intake of high sugar foods such as candy or deserts can cause hyperglycemia. It should be recognized that candy, other sweets, and deserts, not only cause the blood sugar to rise to high levels, but the high sugar levels last until additional insulin is taken.

The Type 2 diabetics are more susceptible to continuous hyperglycemia since they normally do not take insulin. It is next to impossible to drop everything and exercise to reduce the sugar level even if they are smart enough to test their blood sugar when the thirst symptom hits. Without insulin, it is almost impossible to reduce the blood sugar to an acceptable level with exercise alone. Diabetes publications do not explain this risk, and most Type 2 diabetics are unaware that their blood sugar is dangerously high, and they are unable to reduce the level in a timely manner.

The Type 1 diabetic has the tool (insulin) to lower the blood sugar, and most learn to do this automatically, but the Type 2 (without insulin) is unable to lower blood sugar, and often suffers with long-term hyperglycemia.

Another body function known as the dawn phenomenon can cause diabetics high blood sugar in the morning. The dawn phenomenon is when the body produces a supply of hormones in the early morning. All people experience the dawn phenomenon if they are diabetic or not. This is not a serious problem for Type 1 diabetics if they take a long-acting insulin at bedtime, but the Type 2 should be aware of this phenomenon and test his/her blood sugar first thing in the morning.

Hyperglycemia is serious if the condition lasts for long periods. When the body has insufficient insulin to function normally and process the food and glucose into energy for the cells, the body breaks down fats for energy. A waste called ketone results from the fat process, and the body is unable to handle an excess amount of ketones. The ketones build up in the blood and sometimes lead to ketoacidosis, which is life-threatening condition. The symptoms for ketoacidosis are a dry mouth, smelly breath, nausea, and a shortness of breath. Again, the body is telling the diabetic that liquids are required to get rid of the excessive sugar in the blood.

The solution to the insulin intake, hypoglycemia, and hyperglycemia problems is frequent blood sugar testing. The Type 1 diabetic must always check his/her blood-glucose level before each meal to know how much insulin to take, and should frequently check blood sugar between meals. The

Type 2 should also check blood sugar levels before meals to determine the proper meal intake and the exercise required.

Normally the Type 1 diabetic takes a rapid-term insulin before each meal, and since the rapid-term insulin has a four-hour life, it works out that an insulin injection is required before each meal. The amount of rapid-term insulin inserted depends on the sugar level reading at the time of testing and the food to be eaten. If the sugar level is above 100 mg/dl the Type 1 diabetic must mentally calculate the amount of insulin required to reach the 100mg/dl target, and add this amount to the units of insulin required to handle the food. The amount and type food taken dictates the insulin required to handle the food. This again is normally a mental calculation based on the carbohydrates in the food, and the amount of insulin required to handle the glucose in the food.

The test device reading is almost immediate, and is recorded in the device for future reference. However, some diabetics record the sugar reading and the insulin taken on a 3x5 card. This information is needed later in the day when the next meal is taken. The diabetic often forgets the amount of insulin taken and the time of injection, and since insulin overlap is a serious problem, a record of insulin intake is an absolute necessity. The insulin manufacturers provide a paper included with the insulin that shows in graphical form the timing for the insulin action. The insulin curve pictures the onset, peak, and ending timing.

The Type 1 diabetic must calculate the insulin requirements to handle the food intake for each meal. This requires constant and accurate calculations if sugar levels are to be controlled. Most insulin-dependent diabetics store the data in their minds for the average amounts of insulin required to handle their meals. Few go through the mental calculations involving the weight of the food and the number of carbohydrates, and instead "ball-park" the insulin intake requirements based on prior meals. If they pay attention to the results with frequent blood tests, this system works. However, the individual must be rigorous with the blood tests, and not make the assumption that all is good.

Since the insulin inserted is often based on the "ball-park" estimate, or a guess rather than a calculated amount, the diabetic should often check his/her blood-sugar level two hours after a meal. Rapid-term insulin such as Humalog (Eli Lilly) peaks at two hours, and declines to zero after four hours. The blood-sugar level should be approximately 140 mg/gl two hours after a meal. If higher, the Type 1 diabetic may be required to inject additional insulin, but must be careful not to take an amount that could cause an overlap in insulin, and create a hypoglycemic reaction.

The task of remaining between the hypoglycemia and hyperglycemia danger levels is difficult because the range between the two limits is less than 200 mg/gl. Two hours of exercise burns over 100 mg/dl of sugar, and could cause the blood sugar level to reach the hypoglycemia limit. Two candy bars raise the blood sugar over a 100 mg/dl and may cause blood sugar to rise to the hyperglycemia limit. The variables of insulin, food intake, and the diabetic's metabolism are factors in the equation, so remaining between hypoglycemia and hyperglycemia is a difficult task. A Type 1 diabetic must recognize that the limits between low and high blood sugar levels are narrow – approximately 175-200 mg/dl – and manage his/her food intake and insulin intake to avoid hypoglycemia and hyperglycemia. Since each diabetics' metabolism is unique to the individual, it is difficult to use the textbook formulas for the amount of insulin to insert. Trial and error with frequent blood tests is often required to determine the correct amount of insulin.

Frequent blood-glucose tests are necessary to manage diabetes. The diabetic should test in the morning, before each meal, and before going to bed. Occasional blood sugar tests should also be taken during the day to make sure the blood sugar level is under control. If the blood sugar is above the target levels, the Type 1 diabetic must make a correction and take another shot of insulin, and make sure the amount of insulin does not cause an insulin-overlap problem. The only way to control blood sugar is to monitor blood-glucose levels throughout the day. Blood sugar testing is a problem for working people, but is an absolute necessity to avoid hypoglycemia and hyperglycemia. The working diabetic must find time to check his/her blood sugar level during the workday.

The long-term insulin mentioned earlier is necessary for Type 1 diabetics since their pancreas produces no insulin. The long-term insulin produced by some companies lasts for 24 hours and is taken once a day, normally at bedtime. I use Lantus Glargine that is produced by Sanofi-Aventis US located in Bridgewater, New Jersey. Lantus Glargine kicks in about an hour after injection, peaks at 4 hours, and is constant after the peak for the 24 hour period. To avoid hypoglycemia during the night it is necessary to have a blood-glucose level high enough to handle the long-acting insulin. In my case, I take 20 units of Lantus at bedtime and my sugar level must be in the 120-140 mg/dl range to avoid a hypoglycemic reaction during the night. This sugar level was determined by trial and error tests.

RISKS FOR DIABETICS

Diabetes must be controlled and managed if the diabetic is to live a life without complications. Hypoglycemic reactions are serious but the event does warn the individual that sugar is out of control. Hyperglycemia does not cause an immediate reaction in the body but continuous high blood sugar causes ketoacidosis, which is a life-threatening condition. Continuous high blood sugar causes serious effects and the risks are as follows.

- Heart disease – the death rate for diabetics is 1.7 times higher than non-diabetics, and strokes are 1.5 times higher. Heart disease and strokes kill 15 million people every year.

- Foot amputations – high sugar levels cause blood vessel damage that affects the feet.

- Blindness – diabetes is the leading cause of blindness.

- Kidney failure

- Gum disease and loss of teeth

SUMMARY

Diabetics often forget the seriousness of the disease. When an individual lives with diabetes on a daily basis with insulin injections instead of the chemotherapy required with cancer, it is easy to forget how serious diabetes can be.

Diabetics face a difficult challenge in the attempt to manage blood sugar because of the number of variables in the diabetes equation. The life threatening dangers of hypoglycemia and hyperglycemia are always present, so proper management of the disease is an absolute necessity. The Type 1 diabetic can control blood sugar with insulin, but the Type 2 individual has a more difficult time controlling sugar levels since diet and exercise are often avoided. However, both must recognize and pay attention to the risks if sugar level is not managed and controlled. Management of diabetes is possible if the diabetic tests blood sugar levels frequently.

The amount of insulin to take at mealtime is a daily issue for Type 1 diabetics, but the insulin intake is relatively easy if the individual tests for blood sugar regularly. New diabetics are told to begin with a small amount of insulin (four units), and to increase the amount by two units every three days until blood sugar reaches the target level of 140 mg/dl two hours after a meal.

There are many publications listing carbohydrates and calories with suggestions for diets, although many diabetics pay little attention to the recommendations. Diabetics tend to "wing it" and hope for the best.

Research has shown that one unit of rapid-acting insulin handles 15 grams of carbohydrates. However, since each diabetic has a unique metabolism, the diabetic must calculate their individual requirement. The diabetic must test blood sugar levels before each meal to determine the base line, and if the sugar level is above the target of 100 mg/dl, the individual must determine the amount of insulin required to bring the blood sugar down to the target level. This amount is added to the insulin required to handle the meal. The calculation is based on the amount of sugar handled by one unit of insulin. The number of grams of carbohydrates in the meal determines the amount of insulin required to handle the meal. The Type 1 diabetic must be able to calculate this amount, and it is normally done by trial-and-error. The diabetic should then test blood-sugar levels two hours after the meal to make sure the insulin injected handled the meal intake. The Type 2 diabetic has a more difficult time handling meals if the individual is not taking insulin. Managing meals is the key to controlling blood-sugar levels and frequent blood sugar testing is the key to management. The diabetic should always keep in mind that diabetes can be managed, and an almost normal life is possible with proper management.

It is also important to avoid denial because it complicates the situation, and prevents help from family members and business associates. Family members and business associates can often prevent hypoglycemia by recognizing the symptoms, and taking action by recommending that the diabetic take a sugar supplement. In some cases, the hypoglycemia is sudden, and the diabetic is unable to recognize the symptoms. In extreme situations, the diabetic does not recognize hypoglycemia and refuses to take corrective action. In this case, it is necessary for the family member or business associate to immediately call EMT for help. This is a serious problem and not recognized by most diabetic publications.

A diabetic should also wear a medical bracelet or chain around the neck that indicates that the individual is insulin dependent. The medical tag can be useful in case of an emergency because the symptoms of hypoglycemia are similar to drunkenness. The Type 1 diabetic should also carry a sugar pill to counteract the symptoms of hypoglycemia.

After suffering through hypoglycemic reactions for several years, I finally discovered a system for controlling my diabetes. The control and management resulted from years of trial-and-error, but after learning to manage the disease, I have a much-improved outlook on life. My methods for controlling diabetes are the "Ten Commandments for Diabetics."

TEN COMMANDMENTS FOR DIABETICS

1   AVOID DENIAL – ACCEPT THE DISEASE
2   CHECK BLOOD SUGAR BEFORE DRIVING A VEHICLE
3   CHECK BLOOD-SUGAR LEVEL FREQUENTLY
4   DETERMINE THE EFFECT OF ONE UNIT OF INSULIN
5   DETERMINE THE INSULIN REQUIRED FOR MEALS
6   DETERMINE THE LONG-TERM INSULIN REQUIRED
7   AVOID HYPOGLYCEMIA AND HYPERGLYCEMIA
8   CARRY A SUGAR SUPPLEMENT FOR EMERGENCIES
9   MANAGE DIABETES TO 7.0% A1C OR LOWER
10 REASONABLE DIET AND A POSITIVE ATTITUDE

www.ingramcontent.com/pod-product-compliance
Lightning Source LLC
Chambersburg PA
CBHW070758180526
45168CB00004B/1664

Darkroom Photography

The Complete Guide to Mastering the Basics of Darkroom Photography

James Carren

For more books by this author, please visit
www.photographybooks.us

Table of Contents

Introduction

Analog photography is a dying art. When I was in art school and first told that I'd have to take a film photography class, I scoffed. What was the use, I thought, when the entire industry is digital now? Little did I know that some of the most specialized and high-paying jobs that exist are those of people who have the skills to develop film and make darkroom prints. Not only that, but I found that, despite the expense and the hard work required, darkroom was my favorite way to make a photograph.

Darkroom is a science and an art, and it engages your mind in such a way that sitting in front of a computer screen never will, because you get to use your hands and actually watch the chemistry react, watch the image appear right before your eyes. There is something so unique and sacred about that to me.

While this book is mainly meant for those that have never encountered darkroom before and would like to learn the skills, I hope that somewhere in these tips a seasoned photographer might find an alternate way of doing things or an idea that serves them well.

I want to walk through the entire process with you, and give you ideas of how to have resources such as a darkroom where perhaps you currently have none. God knows I've been there.

I'll start from the very beginning: how to select your film and expose it correctly, how to open a film canister, develop the film, and make prints. Then I'll explain how to finish prints and scan the film for digital use, because I feel that it's important to have both versions available to you. I've even included a section on two different types of toners so that you can make your prints stand out just a little bit more.

My goal is to open up the world of film to my generation, so that it continues in its long tradition.

A Quick Rundown on Shooting Film

Shooting film is a little bit different from shooting digital, although if you already have a good, solid foundation, then the principles remain the same. In fact, I have found that most people begin to become great photographers after they have had some experience in the darkroom. The reason for this lies in the fact that analog photography is a much more hands-on process that doesn't provide instant gratification. Therefore, you can't just look at a photograph on a monitor and say, "Oh well that's too bright, let me shoot it again." You have to have a pretty good idea of what you're doing from the start.

Since this book focuses on black and white photography, I would suggest sticking with that. In some respects, color is easier because it's now such a specialized niche that you have to send it off to get it developed. But you also have to make prints digitally, and that's not what this book focuses on.

There are many, many brands of film you can choose from, and it's all up to personal preference. They all perform in generally the same way, but since each film is made by a slightly different process, some are richer than others, some develop more nicely, and some are easier to open. I initially learned on Kodak Tri-X film, but I find it a bit dull in richness and hard to open. I much prefer Kodak T-Max and Ilford Delta. You're never going to know what you like until you shoot it though, so I would suggest creating a little sample pack for yourself to try things out.

ISO also changes things. ISO refers to the speed of your film, or how sensitive to light it is. You probably already know from your digital camera that when you have your ISO set low, like 100 or 200, the sensor lets in a lot less light than if you have it set to 1600. You might also have noticed that pictures taken at low ISOs are much smoother, meaning they have less grain or noise. ISO is all up to a combination of personal preference and light conditions; high ISO is more suitable in low light situations, but you still need to adjust your exposure accordingly. If you are a beginner, or even if you just don't know what you need, start around 400 ISO. It's right smack in the middle of the spectrum and should provide you with good highlights and shadows within a decent spectrum of light.

You'll also have to be meticulous to figure out the correct exposures for things. Try to find nice even light to practice in for your first few rolls, it'll give you a good baseline. Remember that exposure is made up of ISO, aperture, and shutter speed. Shutter speed controls how much movement you see in an image, and aperture controls depth of field, which is how far back you can see into an image.

Also remember that, with film as with digital, if you focus on an area of extreme brightness, your photo will underexpose to compensate and vice versa. To avoid that on your film, you should focus on an area of middle grey to take your reading, then take the photo. It also might be a good idea to try bracketing, which is where you take a photo at the exposure you believe it should be, then close down one stop, and then a second stop, and take a shot at both. You can also do the same going up the scale, although I find that with film, stopping down one or two stops is usually sufficient.

From there, you're ready to go out and shoot.

Prepping Film For Development

After you've shot your film, it's almost time to develop. But if you're working with either 35mm or 120mm, you first have to rewind your film. First, it's important to determine whether or not you have a manual rewind or an automatic rewind. If you have a manual rewind, there will most likely be a crank on top of the camera. Pay attention to the numbers on your camera as you shoot, and keep in mind whether you're shooting a 24 exposure roll or 36 exposure roll. On some rolls of film, you might be able to get more than the expected amount of exposures. This is perfectly okay, but can pose a problem when it comes to storage of negatives. Once you finish your roll of film, you should be able to feel the tension in the camera release a little bit. This means that you've reached the end of your roll of film.

Before you rewind, you should check out your camera's manual and see if there are any special instructions when it comes to rewinding the film. On some cameras, there is a latch at the bottom of the camera that you have to release in order to begin the rewinding process. This is put in place so that you don't accidentally begin to rewind your film as you're shooting. If it's there, release the latch, and begin to wind. You should be able to feel and hear the click of each sprocket as the film is rewound, and the pressure will feel different as you reach the end. Once that pressure releases, it is safe to open the back of your camera. Don't worry if there is a little bit of a film tail sticking out from the canister. If you've rewound it enough, this should just be the end of the film, not an actual exposure, and having the tail sticking out can actually make it easier to get the film out of the canister later.

By nature, an automatic rewind should begin doing its job as soon as you have reached the end of your film. If it doesn't, and you get a few extra exposures, that's no big deal. However, if you don't want these extra exposures, you can check the bottom of your camera to see if there is a recessed button on the bottom. If so, you can use the tip of the pen or pencil to press it and start rewind. Typically, automatic rewind works extremely well, but I did have an instance once where my camera was very old and so the mechanism had broken, causing rewind to stop with about ten exposures to go. If this happens, you might actually be able to hear it, because in the case of my camera, you can hear the motor, and it had begun to sound weak and even stop entirely. Stupid me, I still opened the back of the camera in the light to see what was happening. I would suggest that if you think this might ever be the case with your camera, you take it into a film changing closet or a darkroom before opening the back.

After you're finished rewinding film, it's time to load it onto reels. Pay attention to whether you have 35 or 120mm, because you need a different sized reel for each. And if you happen to have film that is a weird in-between size, be aware that you might have to take a used reel from a roll of film that's already been developed and cut it down so you have something to load it onto.

That aside, I'm going to focus the rest of this chapter and the development chapter using the assumption of 35mm. There are a few things you're going to need in order to load your film and they are: a loading tank, reels, a can opener, and scissors, as well as a loading room or a film change bag. The trick with loading film is that you have to learn to do it by feel because the film cannot be exposed to light or it will be completely ruined (and if even a little light gets in under the door or into the bag, you'll have light leaks or fog on your film, which is fixable in Photoshop, but then you can't make a darkroom print). In order to learn how to do it by feel, I would suggest sacrificing a roll of blank or leaked film to practice on.

You'll also need to decide what kind of reels you'd like to use; there are traditional metal ones and plastic ones. Both work the same, it's just all up to personal preference. I find the plastic ones easier to work with. On your reel, you'll notice two guides, which can either be rectangular or triangular in shape. This is what gets your film onto the track, and you're going to guide your film under them, however, there is a trick to it. We'll get to that in a minute.

You should also decide what kind of tank you want to use. There are myriad brands, but the two I have experience with are Paterson and Jobo. Both are great, but I prefer the Paterson because the water drains out much easier during the rinsing process.

When you're ready to open your film, you'll need to lay out all your things before you shut the door, and put them in an order where you can find everything. You should take the tank apart and set aside the rod, funnel and top. Just a note too . . . even if you're only developing only one roll of film, you should use the correct amount of reels for the tank. It helps with the weight and with making sure you don't get too much developer saturated in the one roll.

After you've shut the door, the first thing you're going to do is open your film canister. Now, this is going to be really easy if you happened to leave some of the tail sticking out. In that case, all you have to do is pull to get it out of the canister, cut the reel, and load it onto the reel. But if you don't have the tail sticking out then you get to experience the joy of using the can opener to get your film out.

There's no right way to do it; you can open it from the top or from the side with the felt-lined lip. You can also use whichever side of the can opener you prefer, although I find that the sharp end works best to fit under either lip. Different brands of film are actually harder to open than others, so just be patient with yourself and realize it'll take some trial and error. You just have to get enough leverage to pop the top off. Even if you just get it up enough to slip the film out, that's good. Just don't scratch the film.

7

After you've got it out of the canister, put your thumb against the attached reel and trim the tail off straight. Also trim the other end, but don't cut too much; you don't want to get into your frames.

To load the film onto the reel, make sure that the guides are facing up and pointing towards your body. Guide the end of the film under the lip, and begin to twist the wheel. Just as with film rewinding, you should be able to feel the film going onto the reel. Keep your fingers on either side as extra guides to make sure the film doesn't pop the track, which it will most likely do the first few times you try this. If you continue to try to roll it after it's popped the track, it'll either fall off onto the floor or will create what's referred to as a kiss, where the film touches itself and leaves a mark.

After you've successfully got the film on the roll, it's time to load your tank. Assuming you're working with a two-reeler, put the rod in the middle of the tank and slide your reels down onto it. Never develop without a rod; this can cause light leaks. Never develop with fewer reels than the tank calls for either; the amount of solution will oversaturate the one roll of film. Put your funnel in and screw it on tight. Before putting the top on and opening the door, turn your tank upside down and shake it to ensure that everything is firmly in place. The last thing you want is your film coming out of the tank before it's fully developed. Now, you're ready to develop.

Processing Film For 35mm and 120mm

To develop 35mm and 120mm film, the process is essentially the same, the only difference will be the type of reels used and the amount of chemistry needed. (It's going to vary dependent on whether you have a 2, 3, or 5 reel tank. Setting up the chemistry is very simple; all you have to do is follow the manufacturer's instructions on the back of the package. Just be very careful when buying your supplies and take note that there is a difference between paper and film chemicals. However, if you want to make a print later, you're going to need both.

I prefer Sprint chemistry because I know it works well with lots of types of paper and film and is, generally speaking, hypoallergenic. Keep in mind that if you choose to use a different brand of chemicals, they might not work well with certain types of paper or film. For example, I have found that Kodak paper developer does not jive well with Ilford paper.

So, what do you need to develop your film, which is the first step on the way to making a print?

You will need:

- Developer
- Stop bath
- Fixer
- Fix remover
- Photo flo

- Access to a sink/running water. Make sure that the water you're using is between 68–72 degrees Fahrenheit. I prefer 68. The cooler the water, the slower the development time, which is good for the film.

To develop your film:

- Mix your developer at a 1:9 ratio with water. (You want more water than developer, make sure you don't get it backwards).

- Get out your other chemicals. Use large beakers and fill them up.

- Start with a one minute pre-rinse of just water on the film. Remember to keep your water between 68–72 degrees. Tap your tank on the sink to remove any existing air bubbles.

- For your developer, start counting the second you pour the chemicals into the tank. Use the instructions based on film type. For example, you might only have to develop for five minutes, or it might be 12, depending on developer and film interaction. Agitate for the first 30 seconds, then for 10 seconds of every minute of development. Agitation ensures that the chemicals are flowing around all of the film, and that the chemicals don't become exhausted.

- As soon as your development time is close to up, start pouring the developer down the sink. Note that developer and photo flo can be safely poured down the drain, but everything else needs to either be stored or disposed of in its own container, which can later be taken away by the proper services.

- Pour in your stop bath. Stop time is a minute and a half. Agitate for the first 30 seconds, as before, and tap to remove air bubbles. Agitate every ten seconds of the remaining minute.

- Next comes fixer for 5 minutes. Agitate as before: constantly for the first 30 seconds then ten seconds of every minute.

- A water rinse is next, to remove the remaining fixer from the film. Fill and dump with clean water 15 times.

- Fix remover comes after the water, for one minute. Agitate every ten seconds

- Do another water rinse, this time 30 repetitions.

- You can now take the funnel out of your tank, pour in photo flo, and spin your reels gently for 15–30 seconds. Dump this, and your film is ready to come off the reel and go into the drying cabinet.

- Some people like to completely take their reels apart to remove the film, although if you just pull gently, you should be fine.

- Leave in the drying cabinet at least half an hour.

- If you don't have access to a drying cabinet, you can also dry your film in a dry shower stall, as this is the cleanest, most dust-free area of the house.

Making Contact Sheets

Here's the materials you're going to need to make a print:

- A pack of RC paper

- A pack of fiber paper

- A contact frame

- A mini site

- An adjustable printing easel

- The correct lens for your film format

- A speed easel

- Some cardboard or an empty paper bag

- Graduated filters

- Canned air

After your film is completely dry, it's time to make contact sheets. Rather than wasting precious fiber paper on contact sheets (because you have to use fiber paper for test strips, which I will explain in a minute) you should use RC paper, or resin coated paper. Resin coated paper is very cheap and slick and is by no means archival, so it shouldn't be used for any final product. However, it is good for just seeing what you have on a film strip.

To make your first contact sheet, you should pick out a roll of film. There's no need to take the negatives out of the sleeve. In fact, if you only have a 24 exposure roll, you'll be able to read the title of the sleeve. Now you have to figure out what exposure the contact sheet needs to be at. Using a piece of cardboard, thick paper, or an empty photo paper bag (the black plastic slip) cover up all but the first strip. This is, of course, after you've got your film properly situated on your paper in the exposure frame. Select a good f/stop, not too large or small. F/11 or 16 is usually best. Expose the first strip for 3 seconds. Move your cover down and expose for 6, and so on until you reach the end of the page.

Now you're going to develop the page. As I said before, I use Sprint chemistry. No matter what chemistry you use, you need to check the manufacturer's instructions for how long to develop, stop, and fix. With Sprint, it's two minutes in developer, 15 seconds in stop, and one minute in fix. Make sure you don't rush through this part . . . it may just be a contact sheet test strip, but you want to make sure it's accurate so that you can determine which photos would be the best to try printing.

After you've developed your test strip, take it out into the light and determine what time you need to expose the contact sheet for. The exposure is correct when you can just barely see the sprockets around the image. You can now go make a contact sheet. Now, even if you shot everything on the same day with the same kind of film, you need to repeat this process for every contact sheet. Run your sheets through the paper dryer, or allow them to air-dry.

Next you want to take your contact sheets and look through them for the great photos. If you are a beginner at darkroom, you need to select photos that have a fairly good tonal range, meaning, good detail in the blacks and highlights that aren't blown out. Later, I'll explain how to fix problems like this, but to make your life easier, it's better to pick a really solidly exposed photo for your first print.

I also like to take my contact sheets in the darkroom to help me out, so mark the photos you want to make with a marker for easy reference.

Making A Basic Print

Don't fall under the misconception that whatever the time for your contact sheet was is the time for your photo. You're going to print final images on glossy fiber paper, for one, which reacts differently, and every photo is also different. Make sure your aperture is set to either f/11 or 16, and put your first negative in the holder. In order to make a good test strip and print, you're going to need to make sure it's in focus. For this, you're going to need your mini site and a sheet of fiber paper. You may want to label the back of this paper with FOCUS SHEET so that you don't accidentally try to print on it. Slide this paper into the speed easel or the adjustable easel, whichever you are using. If you're using an adjustable easel, then you need to adjust the blades to hold your paper and then tape them into place. Also, adjustable easels are much heavier than speed easels so they don't move as much. If you're using a speed easel, you may want to tape the sides down to your workspace.

Slide your focus sheet into place, and put your negative into the negative holder. You have to take it out of the sleeve for this, and it's always a good idea to spray it and the negative carrier off with some canned air first to eliminate dust. You might find that this is tricky the first couple of times, and you might have to fiddle around so you don't have any borders around your image. Next, you need to open your stage and slide the negative carrier into place. The silver knobbies face down and hook into the stage to keep it in place. You should be able to feel it latch if it's properly in place.

Turn on your focus light (without the timer; it should stay on until you turn it off) and adjust the height of the lens up or down until you have your photo at the approximate size you want. Make sure your aperture is open to 2.8 to help you focus, but make sure to adjust it back to a reasonable f/16 or 11 before you begin making test strips or you'll be extremely confused. Eyeball it to get it pretty close to sharp, and then pull out your mini site. Place the magnifier over an area where silver is concentrated (a black part of the image) and look through it. If your photo is in focus, then you should be able to see individual grains. If they look swollen or fuzzy, you need to do some tweaking. You want to do this part without the use of a filter.

After everything's in focus, slide your 2 filter over your negative. You want to make sure it's positioned correctly, otherwise it won't be covering the entirety of the print. Now, you're going to find an area of your photo that has a good tonal range exemplary of the photo as a whole. That's the section where you'll expose your test strip. Turn off your light and cut another piece of fiber paper into at least 5–6 strips. Now, you're going to lay that strip on the part you want, and expose for 3 seconds. Expose the second strip for 6, and so on, then develop them the same way as you did your contact sheet. Take it out into the light, and decide which exposure is the best. This is the exposure you'll use for your basic print.

Now, you're going to expose a whole sheet of paper. Keep in mind that you might want to raise or lower your filter to raise or lower the contrast of the image; 2 is just a starting point.

Seems easy right? But that basic print may not be perfect, and you may have to do it over and over to get the filter and the borders just right. Next, I'm going to teach you some techniques to really make your photo pop.

Dodging, Burning and Other Techniques

After you've made a basic print that you're happy with, take a look at it. Even if the exposure is perfect, does it look exactly how you want it to aesthetically? I'm willing to bet that the answer is probably no. Now you need to figure out what areas of the photograph either need to be lighter or darker. You might be thinking, how do I do this without affecting the entire photograph? This is where the advanced techniques of dodging and burning come into play. Dodging is a technique where you make an area of the photograph look lighter than the original, and burning is where you make an area of the photograph look darker. Typically, you want to do this to make your shadows darker or your highlights pop. Let's start with dodging. Let's say you've figured out that your print needs to be exposed at an f/stop of 8, and an exposure time of 12 seconds, but there's an area of the photo that needs to be considerably lighter. You would take either a piece of cardboard, or a piece of dark plastic, and place it over the area that needs to be lightened. You would then expose your photograph for the amount of time, while keeping the lightening area covered. Now the trick is, you also have to figure out how long that area needs to be covered for. Because it's very unlikely that it needs to be covered for the entirety of that 12 seconds. You'll have to do a test strip for this part as well. Let's say you find that the area needs to be covered for three seconds. You would set your timer for 12 seconds, and cover the area for the first three seconds of that exposure. If you just let your cover lay over the area, you will end up with a very awkward line where you can tell that you tried to dodge. In order to avoid this, you have to constantly move your cover during that three seconds of exposure. These techniques are really hard work, so it will take time to get it right.

Burning works in generally the same way, however, you do your exposure and then you add the amount of time you think the area needs. So in that case, you will expose your image for the full 12 seconds and then add however much time you think you need, covering the rest of the image. Again, it will take some experimentation and test strips to figure out that time, and you have to keep your cover moving to avoid unwanted lines.

It's also entirely possible that you will have both dodging and burning that needs to be done on the same image, so you will have to figure out what order to do it in, and your "dance" (the moving of the cover) for each separate photo.

Aside from traditional dodging and burning, you can also use objects of different shapes directly on top of the paper, to add a collage like element to your work. These are called photograms, and they create an outline of the object on top of whatever image you choose. They can also be an image in their own right.

Toning

There are two types of toners commonly in use for black and white print finishing. By all means, you don't have to tone your finished print, but it can help to add depth to the shadows. Selenium and sepia are the two you'll run into. I'd say that with the current trend in sepia toned filters that you already know that sepia ranges from deep brown to gold. Selenium has more of a purple blue tone to it.

If you do choose to tone your images, you should know that there is some benefit to it. The selenium in particular acts as a protectant and helps make the image more archival. If you want to do this, all you have to do is prepare the selenium bath and dip it in. This won't affect your shadows or highlights at all.

Selenium is also good for just slightly making shadows deeper and richer. It also cools the photo perceptibly.

Sepia is a warming toner, and can range from very subtle yellow in the highlights to a deep brown overall.

Experiment with different times for soaking the print, and different concentrations of the toner to get different results. Label the back of your prints and keep a record of them to refer back to later.

Final Print Preparation

By this point, your prints are probably hanging out in the water bath. As I stated in the chapter on making prints, it's best to let them wash in moving water for 20–30 minutes. Next, you're going to put them in a tray with enough paper fixer remover to cover them, and for the next 5–10 minutes, you need to shuffle the prints through the chemistry. This will remove any excess chemistry that might still be caught in the paper, and the shuffling keeps fresh chemistry moving over the paper so that it doesn't become exhausted.

After you're done with the fixer remover, it's time to put your images in the archival wash. You should leave the prints there for at least 20 minutes, though you can leave them up to an hour. I wouldn't suggest any longer than that though, because otherwise the emulsion can begin to peel away from the paper.

When you get them out, they have to be squeegeed to remove the excess water, otherwise they'll never dry, and will be more susceptible to rack marks. Do the front and the back, and be firm but gentle. The last thing you want is to rip a finished print, and believe me, it happens.

Finally, you want to put your images on a drying rack. Make sure they're spaced out enough to not touch, because they will stick together and rip. Some people like to dry their images face up to avoid rack marks, but again, if they've been wrung out enough, this shouldn't really be an issue. I don't like to dry images face up because if there are images on the rack above, you get water drips on your images. You also get a lot of dust, which is a pain in the neck to remove.

Leave your images there at least for the night. In the morning they'll have to be heat pressed to remove the curling. If you are using a traditional heat press, you can stick the prints directly into the press, although if you're worried about burning you can always place them, stacked, in between two pieces of cardboard. Alternatively, if you don't have access to a heat press, you can use a dry iron with cardboard over the image to protect it. I find that it takes about two minutes to press about five images altogether.

Your prints are now ready for matting and framing.

Making Scans and Developing Digitally

Some people like to make direct scans of the images they've made, and while that's fine and it works, I find that scanning the film produces a better quality image. I learned how to scan on an Imacon scanner, but those are very expensive and unless you go to school for photography or have the extreme luck to have access to a studio that has one, you'll probably have to use a flatbed scanner. That works just fine, but if you're buying one of your own, I would suggest an Epson flatbed that's made for film so that you also get the film scanning kit with it. The film scanning kit comes with a 4x5, 120mm, and 35mm magnetic holder that makes it much easier to hold the film still.

Every scanner is different, so I'll just provide some generalized guidelines for the Imacon and general flatbed scanners.

First things first, when you scan, you should come prepared with gloves, canned air, and an anti-static cloth. Wipe down your work area and spray it off to get rid of as much dust as you can beforehand. This leads to less cleanup in post. Make sure your film strip lines up with the magnetized holder, otherwise the scan will be off. Clipping it in can be finicky, so just do it again if the Imacon doesn't want to cooperate. Go into the Flextight program and open it up. The first thing you want to do to prep is to turn off the sharpening on the image. Then you need to select the type of film that you have and the ISO from the dropdown menu. In this case, you want to make sure that the type you select also reads negative, otherwise the machine thinks your negative is a positive. Then set your ppi to a high resolution, especially if you want to print them large later. Be careful though; if you change your format or film type, the resolution also resets to 300, so just be sure to double check things before you hit scan. You should see a preview, then you'll be asked to name your final scan.

So that's all the technical, but what about edits? Many people, when they first learn to scan, mistakenly believe that you should edit your photo to look like you want the finished product to. But I'm here to tell you that this scan is like your master copy, your RAW file, and your job here is not to make it look aesthetically pleasing, but to capture as much information from the film as you can. This often means tamping down highlights that you really want to be brighter, and lifting shadows you want to be deep and dark. Make sure you can see every detail of the image, and that you're as close to a proper exposure as is possible. Generally, one film strip is going to be fairly similar in exposure so you should be able to make generalized corrections to the entire strip. However, if you do find that you have an outlier or that the photos need some individual tweaking, you can select it and only edit that picture.

The end result of this process is going to look very grey and unappealing, but I promise you it will give you the best image to edit in Photoshop or Lightroom.

If you have to use a flatbed scanner, just make sure that you have a way to secure the negatives if you don't have the film holders, and make sure that it's set on Professional mode at a reasonably high ppi. I would say at least 600.

Now, you can bring your scans into Photoshop and clean them up. If you haven't made darkroom prints yet, I would suggest doing this part first, especially if you plan on using advanced darkroom techniques. This way, you can experiment without wasting paper. Figure out what aesthetic you want and do it on the digital copy. Take notes for what you would have to do to get it to correspond in the darkroom. It will make your life much easier.

Conclusion

It is my hope that you are now more confident in the art of darkroom photography. If this is a brand new foray for you, hopefully you are more excited than overwhelmed, and curious about stepping into a darkroom. Now you know how to set up your own darkroom, and make a photograph from start to finish.

Once you've mastered the basics of how to develop your film, begin to experiment with the contrast to see if you find a style you like better. The same goes for the actual prints. Once you've learned how to make a good, solid, basic print on glossy paper, begin to experiment with the dodging and burning techniques I go through in chapter 8. Learn to fully express yourself through your prints and find all the possibilities you can in your images.

Learning analog can be a frustrating and long journey, but if you're truly passionate or curious about learning it, make sure you stick with it, because it's very rewarding. Even if you find that it's not your thing, I hope that you will at least learn the basics. I say this because doing analog makes you much more meticulous. Mistakes are much harder to correct, so it's better to get it right with each step you take. And the more careful you are, the better quality your final image will be. Even if you go back to digital completely, you'll find that your work gets much stronger after learning some darkroom skills. This is because you learn to be much more meticulous about each step you take, and thus have a higher standard of quality for yourself. You also end up having less work to do in post.

So as you begin your journey, take your time, be patient with yourself, be willing to experiment and make mistakes, and have fun.